STROKE RESTORATION

STROKE RESTORATION

Functional Movements for Patients and Caregivers

with
Illustrations of Progressive Exercises

by
Yaffa Liebermann
Physical Therapist
Geriatric Clinical Specialist

Illustrations by Kate Soko

Prime Rehabilitation Services, Inc.

ISBN 978-0-692-00081-6

Cataloguing-in-Publication data for this book is available from the Library of Congress (LC Control No. 2008934592).

Published by Prime Rehabilitation Services, Inc.
P.O. Box 785
Oakhurst, NJ 07755
(732) 493-3100
Fax (732) 493-4285
www.primerehab.com
info@primerehab.com

Contents

Publisher's Note

This book is not intended to be a substitute for the advice of a physician, physical therapist, occupational therapist, or speech language pathologist. Readers who suspect they may have specific medical problems should consult a physician about any of the suggestions included in this book. The information in the book is not all inclusive, and it focuses on some therapy aspects of stroke treatment.

The author has made every effort to ensure the accuracy of the information herein, particularly with regard to techniques and procedures. However, appropriate information sources should be consulted before initiating any exercise. The author, editors, and publishers cannot be held responsible for any errors found in the book.

Under no circumstances—including, but not limited to, negligence—will the publisher or its members, affiliated entities, employees, directors, agents, or any other parties involved in the creation, production, or delivery of this book be liable for any direct, indirect, incidental, special, consequential, or punitive damages that result from using this information.

STROKE RESTORATION

Introduction

The medical term for stroke is cerebral vascular accident, or CVA. This means that either (a) the blood supply to part of the brain is shut off or (b) there is bleeding within the brain. It is, in essence, a brain "attack" that results in a brain "injury." In a brain attack, some brain cells are permanently destroyed, while others temporarily do not function due to brain swelling. As the brain heals, the swelling goes down and the cells in the swollen area begin to function again. The consequences of a brain attack are different for each patient; therefore each regains his strength and movement in different ways. The severity of the CVA and amount of time since the CVA occurred as well as the patient's age, medical condition, attitude, and perseverance to push forward will affect overall recovery.

A stroke may be frightening to both patient and family, since they all find themselves in unfamiliar territory. A patient may do well with one activity, but have trouble with another seemingly easier task. Those who have had a stroke often demonstrate weakness on one side of the body or difficulty moving, swallowing, talking, or thinking. It is comforting to know that stroke patients usually have at least some natural healing, continue to restore their movement in rehabilitation, and then continue to improve through practicing at home. Stroke survivors should realize that some function may never return, therefore hope and realization should intertwine with each other.

I am a physical therapist, geriatric clinical specialist, and chief executive officer of Prime Rehabilitation Services, Inc. The purpose of writing this book is to help caregivers teach stroke patients how to regain strength and restore functional movement so that they will be able to take care of their own daily needs—such as dressing, bathing, eating, and walking. The information in this book can be applied to anyone who has suffered from a disease or event that's weakened the body, leaving them unable to perform as they did before. The illustrations demonstrate several techniques of care; they show patients how to move and show caregivers how to support patients, providing ideas for progressive functional treatments for professionals (physical, occupational, and speech therapists).

The book relates primarily to a brain attack that affects the strength and sensation of one side of the body, and it focuses on a few basic aspects of body motion:

- **Trunk control** – Stabilization, strength, and flexibility for the body's core structure, followed by arm and leg movements
- **Weight shifting** and equal weight bearing on both sides of the body
- **Correct breathing** – Long exhalation (in flexion) versus short inhalation (in extension)
- **Repetition** – The best way to increase brain plasticity (its ability to change) and restore motion

Note: In this book, I refer to the patient as "he" or "him." The words "family" and "caregiver" are used for the people who take care of the patient at home or in a facility; I refer to the family member or caregiver as "she" or "her." I do not intend to imply that all patients are male or that all caregivers are female. This simply makes my writing—and your reading—a little easier.

Effects of a Stroke

Some of the common effects of a stroke are as follows:

- Lack of awareness, or ignoring things, on one side of the body
- Weakness or paralysis on one side of the body
- Difficulty with balance and coordination
- Difficulty walking and transferring from a bed to a chair or from a chair to the toilet
- Difficulty with speech
- Difficulty with vision on the weakened side
- Pain, numbness, or odd sensations
- Difficulty with memory, thinking, attention, or learning
- Difficulty swallowing
- Difficulty with bowel or bladder control
- Getting tired very quickly
- Sudden bursts of emotion, such as laughing, crying, or anger
- Mood changes and depression

Getting the Most Out of Rehabilitation

The rehabilitation team in sub-acute nursing homes typically consists of doctors, nurses, physical therapists, occupational therapists, speech language pathologists, and social workers. After discharge from the hospital, caregivers and patients become an integral part of the restoration process of increasing function. The team has regular meetings to discuss the patient's condition and progress. They all focus and work together to meet the treatment goals.

If you are a stroke survivor in rehabilitation, be a partner in your care. Record important information about your treatment and progress, and write down any questions you may have. Know that you are the most important person in your treatment.

Patients should do the following:

- Make sure others understand that you want to be involved in making decisions about your care. State your wishes and opinions on matters that affect you.
- Bring your questions and concerns to the team meetings.

Caregivers should do the following:

- Encourage the patient to participate in rehabilitation, and help him practice skills learned in therapy.
- Ask to attend some of the rehabilitation sessions. This is a good way to learn the exercises and the best way to support the patient when moving.

Caregivers *and* patients should do the following:

- Participate in education offered for stroke recovery. Join a stroke support group. Look up information on the Internet. Read magazines and books about strokes.

Many patients find that rehabilitation is hard work. They discover that maintaining function while working to regain movement is challenging. It is normal to feel tired and discouraged at times, because tasks that used to be easy before the brain attack are now difficult. The important thing is to notice the progress made and feel pride in each incremental achievement.

Be Aware of the Weak Side

One of the consequences of stroke is that the patient is unaware of and ignores one side of the body. Therefore, it is important for the caregiver to be aware of the weak side.

Keep these tips in mind:

- Position the bed in the hospital/nursing home so that the patient's weak side faces the door and he can watch outside activity—people walking, food being delivered by kitchen personnel, medication being given by nurses, and so on. This position stimulates sensation and awareness of the weak side.

- As the caregiver approaches the patient, she needs to stand in front of the patient so he can see and identify the visitor. Once recognized, the visitor can move to the weak side.

- Visitors can sit on the patient's weak side and lightly touch his arm or hand. This allows the visitor's positive energy to flow to the patient while engaging in activities such as playing cards, watching television, listening to the radio, or playing a board game.

- Caregivers should move the weak limb as often as possible, as instructed by a therapist, to alleviate pain and maintain full movement in the joints to prevent stiffness.

- When the patient progresses, he will be able to move the weak arm by himself, using the strong arm to help.

Precautions for Caregiver Before and During Exercises

Before Exercises

Before performing any exercises with the patient, be sure to do the following:

- Check with the therapist to verify that any new exercises are appropriate.
- Carefully review the pictures to see the direction in which to perform the movement.
- Before performing any standing activity from a wheelchair, make sure the wheels are locked.

During Exercises

During exercises with the patient, be sure to do the following:

- Be gentle when holding the arm or leg.
- Do not force a movement. When you feel that the movement does not flow well, stop and check the reason for the limitations.
- Work slowly, and allow the patient to perform at his own pace.
- Repeat the exercise three to five times in each session. This allows the muscles and joints to become familiar with the movement.
- Practice the exercise on both sides of the body equally.

- Remind the patient to use the weak side.
- Gradually reduce the amount of assistance provided. You want to support the patient and help when he is weak. As function returns, muscles can then take over performing the task.
- Be positive, and ask the patient to perform small tasks—and emphasize any achievements, small as they may seem. Unsuccessful movement tends to frustrate the patient—while success, even with assistance, is encouraging and fulfilling.
- Your goal is to find out what the patient is capable of doing alone, what he can do with help, and what his limitations are. Avoid doing things for the patient that he is capable of performing independently. Each time he achieves a movement, his confidence will grow.

Knowing When to STOP

When you work with a patient, check his vital signs and use parameters set by his physician. You need to know when to STOP.

Look for these signs:

- If the patient's breathing becomes too heavy or too rapid—STOP, let him rest, and/or notify the nurse.
- If the patient starts to perspire too much—STOP, let him rest, and/or notify the nurse.
- If the patient suddenly becomes weak—STOP, let him rest, and/or notify the nurse.
- If the patient becomes pale or bright red—STOP, let him rest, and/or notify the nurse.
- If the patient becomes very frustrated—STOP, let him rest, and try a less challenging exercise.

Communication: Speech Evaluation and Treatment

A speech language pathologist (SLP) can help if the patient has difficulties after the brain attack with communication—listening, reading, understanding, processing, or expressing needs. The SLP will teach the family the best way to communicate with the patient. Patients can get depressed when they realize they have suddenly lost control of their lives and other people are making decisions for them. This is why an early intervention from an SLP is crucial. The SLP will analyze the patient's ability to understand and the patient's obstacles to talking, and then guide the caregivers accordingly.

A patient may suffer from one of these:

- **Receptive Aphasia** – Difficulty processing information, following directions, or identifying common objects. The patient is very confused and does not understand what people ask him to do. He needs more time than usual to process what he is told.

- **Expressive Aphasia** – Difficulty communicating and expressing oneself. The patient cannot find the right words or put the words in a logical order. He might understand what people say and want to reply correctly, but the words do not come out of his mouth the way he wants. Sometimes he might repeat one word—for example, say "no, no, no" even if he means "yes."

Here are some ideas for the caregiver about how to communicate with the patient:

- Speak in a normal voice—do not scream.
- If it is very difficult for the patient to hear you from the weak side, talk to the good side.
- Ask simple yes-or-no questions.
- Speak slowly and clearly, and give the patient enough time to reply.
- Ask the patient to repeat the sentence if you do not understand him.
- Ask the patient to practice saying words out loud.

Dysphagia: Difficulty Swallowing

The other issue that is crucial from the beginning of the brain attack is food intake. The patient may have lost muscle strength not only in an arm and leg, but also in the mouth and throat. This can make it difficult to swallow as well. Food might go down the "wrong tube," into the lungs instead of the stomach, causing aspiration pneumonia.

If a patient shows signs of aspiration (coughing, throat clearing, or a "gurgle" vocal quality), the SLP may restrict the patient from a certain food consistency (e.g., thin liquids) and recommend a **modified barium swallow** to rule out aspiration. Modified barium swallows are also done in the absence of signs of aspiration when patients have documented vocal fold paralysis or frequently occurring pneumonia of unknown origin—particularly if they have a neurology history, like a stroke. The barium swallow is primarily a structural evaluation of the entire esophagus (the swallowing tube); it can rule out narrowing of the passage, tumors, obstruction, etc. The radiologist typically comments on some aspects of esophageal structures, such as contractures (shortening or tightening of muscles or tendons). The test helps the SLP assess the swallowing ability and food consistency.

Diet is established and adjusted by the SLP and dietitian. For safety reasons, the patient should chew food on the strong side of his mouth. The patient should not try to chew on his weak side until both he and the caregiver are trained by the speech language pathologist.

The SLP may give other instructions such as these:

- Caregivers can sit by the patient's weak side for aware-ness.
- For safe swallowing, patients can sit with the hips at a 90-degree angle.
- To prevent aspiration, patients should try to keep the chin tucked in.
- Patients should stay seated for thirty minutes after eat-ing or drinking.
- Patients should take small bites of food at each meal.
- Patients can alternate solids and liquids.
- Patients should take extra swallows for safety.

Correct Breathing

The stroke patient may suffer from shortness of breath due to overall weakness. The therapist can prepare the patient to cope with stressful situations by teaching him how to breathe properly. It is important that the patient practices breathing when not under physical stress. This way, when the patient experiences shortness of breath during a stressful activity—such as walking or climbing stairs—the body is trained to overcome the difficult situation. The goal is to concentrate on breathing while directing the patient's mind away from the difficult task and, at the same time, gaining more oxygen to the lungs.

Long Exhalation (Breathing Out) Versus Short Inhalation (Breathing In)

Exhalation is a forced movement of the body, while inhalation is an automatic movement. Long and deep exhalations are necessary to clear the lungs and make room for oxygenated air. The best way to practice breathing is by exhaling twice as long as inhaling. For example, have the patient breathe out for a count of six, and breathe in for a count of three (a two-to-one ratio). Caregivers can help by massaging the upper muscles of the patient's shoulders and releasing the tension of his body so that air can easily flow in and out.

Flexion (Bending Forward) Versus Extension (Straightening Up)

The patient should exhale (breathe out) during flexion (bending) of the trunk—in other words, when he bends over. The patient should inhale (breathe in) during extension of the trunk—or when he stands up straight again. He can practice breathing out when bending his body forward to reach for a cup of water, and breathing in when expanding his chest and straightening back up to drink the water.

The caregiver can help by putting one hand on the patient's sternum (upper chest) to create light pressure upon exhalation (breathing out). This helps the patient breathe out.

Adaptive Devices

Many different types of adaptive devices and durable medical equipment are available to assist the patient in becoming more independent. Need is determined by the type and level of the patient's functional deficits and by the patient's ability to adjust to those deficits. Using a device should not substitute for reasonable efforts to teach the patient a method to perform the task. The device may serve as a useful supplement. However, it should be discontinued if the adapted method cannot be learned, requires too much effort, or increases frustration for the patient or caregiver.

The patient and family should be involved in selecting adaptive devices and should be trained in their use. Since some of these devices are expensive, the patient's financial situation and insurance coverage also need to be explored.

Splinting

When a joint is flaccid (loose or limp), swollen, or contracted, the therapist has to decide if a splint is appropriate to support the joint. The splint may be temporary or permanent. The therapist evaluates the patient and treats him a few times prior to establishing a splint schedule. She can study the patient's behavior and assess whether he will tolerate the splint or take it off shortly after application. The therapist may continue to provide skilled care—by checking, adjusting, and ensuring a proper fit and proper amount of time to apply the splint—before transferring the care of the splint to the family or to restorative nursing.

Goals of a Splint

Splints are usually applied to achieve one or more of the following:

- Promote skin integrity (make sure skin is free of irritation).
- Maintain and/or increase movement in the joint.
- Allow for adequate hygiene.
- Decrease pain in the joint.
- Prevent increased contractures (tightening of muscles).
- Decrease edema (swelling) in the arm or leg.

Treatment Approach

The therapist should evaluate the patient and decide how to

proceed with the splint utilization:

- Determine the appropriate splint to use, and adjust it as needed.
- Establish a schedule for wearing the splint, and monitor skin integrity (for irritations).
- Develop a restorative program. The nursing staff will be in charge of applying the splint per the therapist's advice.
- Train the patient, facility staff, and family on the importance of stretching the joint slowly prior to applying the splint.

Wheelchair Management

During the early stages of patient recovery, he might benefit from using a wheelchair. The family should encourage him to propel the wheelchair unassisted. When visiting the patient, family members should not push the wheelchair from the back, but instead help as needed on the weak side. This achieves two goals: (a) the patient can see and interact with the family and facility staff and (b) moving the wheelchair independently will stimulate the muscles of the entire body, especially those of the weak side.

It will provide the patient freedom to travel safely in the facility, go to the bathroom, and participate in activities with others. The patient can propel the wheelchair in different ways, in accordance with his ability:

- The patient can use his strong hand to turn the wheel on the strong side, as the strong leg pushes and pulls the chair along the floor in the desired direction.

- While placing the weak arm on the arm rest and the weak leg on the foot rest, the patient can use both legs as pushing, pulling, and steering devices. The movement of the feet connects the body to the ground. The patient can gain a better sense of the change in the floor surface so that when he walks, gait adjustment can increase safety.

- The patient can stomp his feet on the floor when he sits. This helps him gain muscle strength, stability, and safety awareness. He can do this while reading, talking on the phone, using a computer, or watching TV.

Trunk Control

A stroke patient who has lost strength in the arm and leg on one side has most likely also lost strength in his trunk muscles on the same side. Therefore, the status of the muscle function has changed and presented itself in a different way: the two sides of his body are divided into two halves, and there is no interplay between the good side and the affected side. The strong side of his back and his abdominal muscles used to get signals from the other side; these signals would tell them which way to act in order to keep the body in a straight position. Due to the brain attack, the signals have now vanished, and the strong side has to compensate for the lost function of the weak side.

Research shows that the trunk is controlled not only by the motor and sensory cortex of the brain, but also by other vital areas, like the cerebellum and mid-brain. Therefore, if one little segment is destroyed, temporarily or permanently, there are enough cells remaining in the brain to take over the action and produce a motion.

Trunk rotation, balance in sitting, balance in standing—all of these movements prepare the body's core structure to get stronger, and they allow a good base for the arms and legs to function.

Weight Bearing/Weight Shifting to the Weak Side

Weight bearing, or weight shifting, are successful ways for the patient to regain movement. The stroke survivor tends to stand more on his strong leg and use his strong arm. So he should try to shift weight onto his weak leg and actively use or lean passively on his weak arm.

Bearing the patient's weight on both legs accomplishes the following:

- Normalizes tone – increases low tone and decreases high tone
- Provides normal movement experience – patient learns the correct motion from the strong side and relates it to the weak side
- Provides normal sensory experience
- Allows energy to flow from the strong leg and arm to the weak leg and arm

The exercises in this book demonstrate shifting weight onto the weak leg, which sometimes suffers from a lack of deep feeling. The intent is to practice shifting weight in various positions—for example, holding onto the parallel bars, holding onto a stable table, holding onto a heavy sofa, and holding onto a kitchen counter.

While sitting, the patient can stomp his feet on the floor during reading, talking on the phone, or watching television. By connecting to the floor, he can better sense the change in floor surface so that when he walks, he can adjust his gait to the changing surface to increase his safety.

During transfers, the patient should shift his trunk weight forward as he bends, aligning his nose with his knees, then place his hands on the armrests to push up from the wheelchair.

Transfers: Sitting to Standing, Wheelchair to Bed

When a patient changes position from sitting to standing, he needs all his muscle strength. Transferring requires much more muscle power than walking. Therefore, the patient may need help from more than one person to stand up, while needing the assistance of only one person to walk.

Preparation for Transfers – Rocking

It is helpful for the patient to rock backward and forward before changing positions. This motion makes the trunk flexible, and it prepares the body for the direction of the movement while gathering momentum for the transfer. It also connects the caregiver to the patient through holding hands and transferring energy to each other.

Shifting Body Weight

Place the patient's head in the opposite direction from where his buttocks will go. Move his head forward, and place his nose in line with his knees (over his toes), so that his buttocks goes up. This shifts away part of his weight and lightens the load over his buttocks for a smoother transfer.

Transfer Steps

To transfer the patient from the wheelchair to the bed, the caregiver should do the following:

1. Position the wheelchair at a 45-degree angle to the bed.
2. Lock the wheelchair's brakes.
3. Remove the patient's feet from the footrests, and either remove the footrests or swing them out of the way. If needed, remove the armrest that is next to the bed.
4. Make sure the patient's feet are flat on the floor.
5. Position yourself in front of the patient's feet, and place your knees against the patient's knees.
6. Lean the patient forward and away from the bed.
7. Reach around the patient's shoulder with your arm that is closest to the bed, and grasp his belt or waistband.
8. Hold the patient's trunk—do not grasp onto the patient's arm.
9. Put your other arm in front of the patient's opposite shoulder to prevent him from falling forward.
10. Help the patient transfer from the wheelchair onto the bed by leading the movement with his hips.

Walking

When the caregiver helps the patient walk, she should stand on the patient's weak side and support his trunk while guiding him. The patient should shift weight onto one leg before lifting the other leg.

The best way for the patient to begin walking is to simplify the process into several steps:

1. Move the walker.
2. Move the strong leg.
3. Shift weight onto the strong leg.
4. Shift weight onto the arms and hands, which lean on the walker to share the support.
5. Move the weak leg forward, preferably past the strong leg.
6. Shift weight onto the weak leg.
7. Repeat.

Using Walkers

Using a walker is a safe way to provide stability for the patient (walkers are preferable to canes). Some patients view the walker as a symbol of weakness and therefore refuse to use it. However, using a walker can be extremely beneficial to the patient while he is regaining the use of his weak side. Holding the walker with the hand and putting weight on the leg cause an increase of deep sensation, which promotes faster restoration.

When foot muscle (dorsiflexor) strength does not return after a stroke, and the foot does not clear the floor, the therapist can measure the patient for a brace (ankle-foot orthotics, or AFO) to keep the toes off the floor when advancing the leg forward. It is better to have a brace with a hinge in the ankle joint to allow movement. A one-piece, off-the-shelf brace might stimulate, and increase, the plantar flexor muscles' tone and interfere with push-off.

Repetition

The brain attack has left the patient with one weak side, but it has also confused the strong side, which has to relearn all of its movement. The strong side now has to perform double the action—the regular movement it performed before the stroke, plus extra work to take over for the weak side. The patient cannot learn this quickly, nor can he actively follow quick movement. The therapist and patient have to continue to practice and persevere in the face of slow progress. The patient needs more time than usual to understand the process and perform a movement.

Repetition is the key. Whatever the patient is able to achieve in one session, he usually regresses by 75% the next day. The therapist has to reintroduce the movement so that the patient relearns the motion and reestablishes the muscle memory. At least five repetitions of a movement in one session help the patient better remember it.

The physical therapist can practice transfers from the wheelchair to the bed, while the occupational therapist can practice transfers from the wheelchair to the toilet. Each transfer is different for the patient, so he needs to practice in all the different settings to prepare for regular home situations.

The repetition helps the plasticity of the brain (its ability to change) and its recovery potential. Repetition "unmasks" relatively inactive pathways, helps undamaged brain tissue take over functional representation, connects synapses that were never connected before, and stimulates neuron cells to be active in a new capacity.

In sub-acute nursing homes, therapists invest time and effort teaching the family, nurses, and nurses' aides in correct bed mobility, transfers, walking patterns, activities of daily living (ADL), talking, and swallowing. The constant repetition of exercises helps remind the patient's muscles of the proper movement. It is important for all caregivers to perform each activity in the same way. Then the patient can memorize movements and not get confused by different techniques for the same motion.

Returning Home

If the stroke survivor does not succeed in getting all of his muscles to a regular functioning level, he is going to lag behind when he goes home. There is going to be an adjustment period for the patient and the entire family. Life has changed, but it must go on in a different way. There will be adjustments to jobs, home environment, social life, and travel habits—not to mention an entirely different approach to married life. Suddenly, the patient must be fully dependent on another family member—while prior to the brain attack, the patient was an independent person and the family counted on him.

There are endless scenarios of life changes, but from my observation, most stroke survivors and their families have overcome the hurdles well. If a social life used to end at 8:00 pm, and after the stroke attack it ends earlier at 6:00 pm, that is an easy change. If traveling before the stroke meant going overseas, but now the travel is not farther than one hour away, that's an easy change. If someone has to drive the stroke patient to work for the first few months, that's an easy change. People like to help. Family and friends can change their schedules to lend a helping hand. The most important thing is for the patient to stay in high spirits and not give up when muscle strength does not return as quickly as he would like it to.

Researchers are always finding more ways to achieve additional progress after a brain attack. The stroke survivor should continue to strive to achieve more movements. Research is not giving up on the mystery of the mind and its ability to recover, so neither should the patient. He has to push himself to allow re-mapping in the brain that will result from practicing progressive functional exercises.

The patient should be regularly checked by a doctor. If the hand does not function properly, then a skilled occupational therapy intervention is needed. If the leg is not holding the body well, a skilled physical therapy intervention is needed. And if speech or swallowing is problematic, the skilled care of a speech language pathologist is needed. It is very beneficial to seek help from a skilled therapist to see if there is a new approach or new exercises to stimulate different muscles.

If insurance does not cover therapy services because the carrier does not think functional ability will change, the patient should contact the provider and explain his limitation and its obstacles to regular life activities. He should try to receive approval for at least ten sessions at a time. The patient himself should take this responsibility and not expect others to organize doctor and therapist visits.

Laughter is something we forgot to use as a tool for recovery and a happy existence. More and more research has demonstrated that laughter, prayer, and positive energy are keys to a healthy life. They build the immune system and help fight disease. Cheer up by laughing more often, remembering nice things that have happened in the past, listening to music that appeals to you, and directing energy and thought to a creative path. All of that can have an effect on the body for relaxing and diffusing stress. Choose a hobby that is challenging and fulfilling, and make your body move.

Closing Remarks

I hope this book will be a source of help to patients who have experienced decreased body functionality and to their families. In order to regain the level of function that he had prior to the brain attack, the patient should keep practicing weight-bearing motions. One day, a stronger and smoother movement will develop—and sometimes, hopefully, full recovery will prevail.

Love the patient and listen to him!
Hug him and praise him!
You can make a change!
You are the most important support he can have!

Illustrations of Progressive Exercises

Feeding from the Weak Side

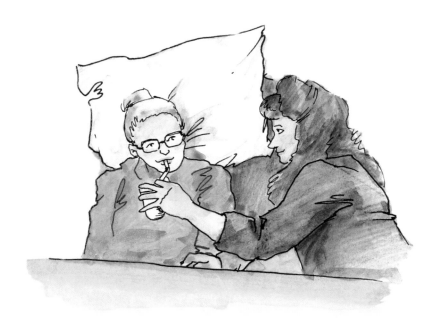

Patient: Sit upright at a 90° angle.

Caregiver: Give the patient a drink, and help the patient eat while sitting on the weak side, as instructed by the speech language pathologist (SLP).

Correct Breathing – 1

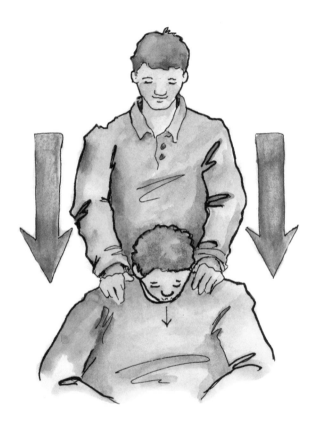

Patient: Breathe out twice as long as you breathe in (a ratio of 2 to 1).

Caregiver: Help by lightly massaging the upper muscles of the patient's shoulders.

Correct Breathing – 2

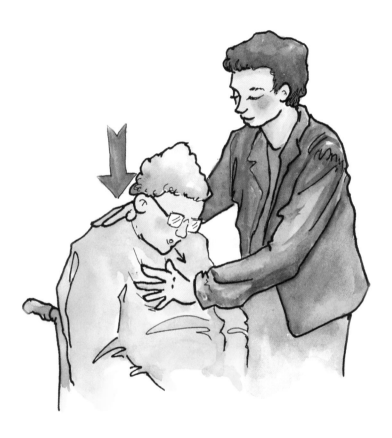

Caregiver: Help the patient breathe out when bending the body forward. Put light pressure on the patient's chest and shoulders to guide the movement.

Preparing to Use a
Bed Pan and Dressing

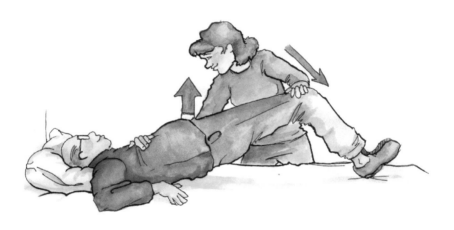

Caregiver: Bend both of the patient's knees, and press down lightly for stability.

Patient: Lift up your buttocks.

Preparing to Sit Up

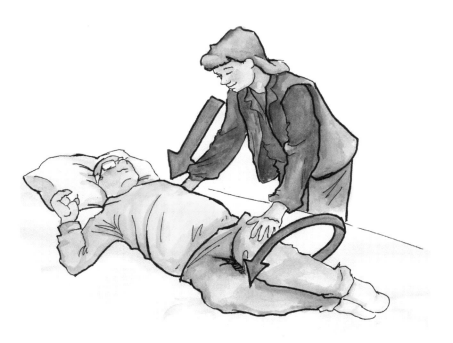

Caregiver: Put your hands on the patient's shoulder and knee to
gently provide proper guidance.

Patient: Bend your knees, and move them together from side
to side.

41

Reducing Spasticity in the Arm

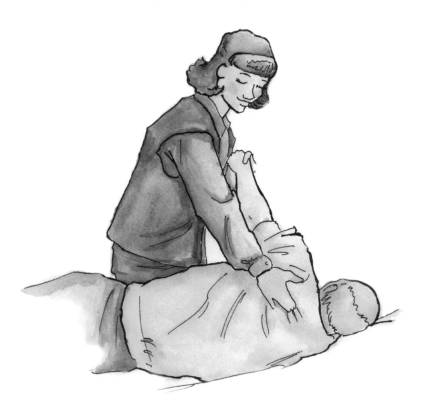

Patient: Lie down on your strong side, and keep your weak/spastic arm on top. Move the arm forward.

Caregiver: Hold the patient's weak hand for support, and keep the elbow straight. Put your other hand on the patient's shoulder blade, and gently pull forward.

Caring for a Spastic Hand

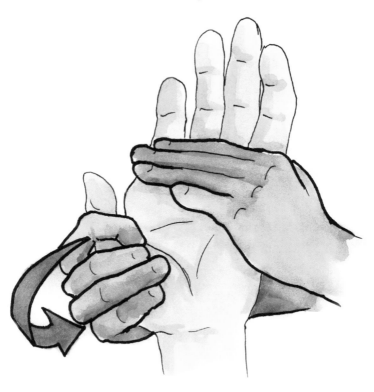

Caregiver: Slide your hands into the palm of the patient's hand, and stretch it to open slowly.

Getting Out of Bed – 1

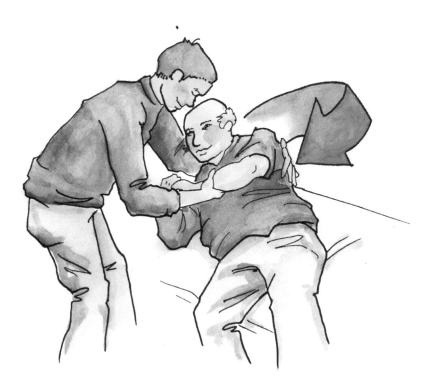

Caregiver: Help turn the patient's body in a circular movement.
Patient: Push up from the bed with your elbow.

Getting Out of Bed – 2

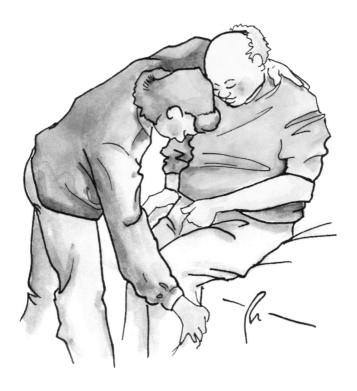

Caregiver: Support the patient's body, and position the legs.

Patient: Push with your hand to reach the sitting position.

Weight Bearing on Elbow and Shoulder

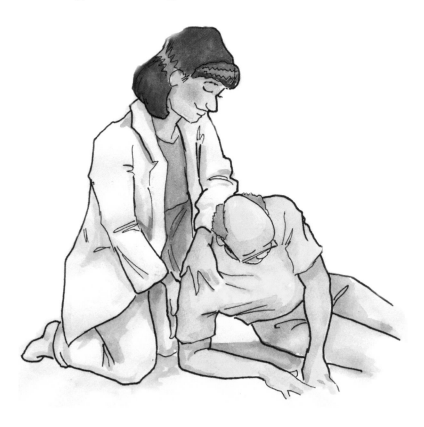

Caregiver: Stabilize the patient's shoulder from the back and front.

Patient: Move your body backward and forward.

Self Weight Bearing on Elbow and Shoulder

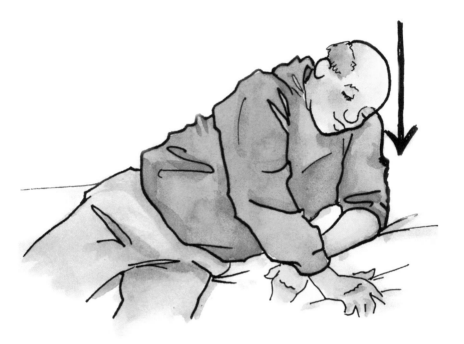

Patient: Lean on your elbow and shoulder. The weight bearing stimulates a flaccid arm while decreasing tone in a spastic arm.

Weight Shifting

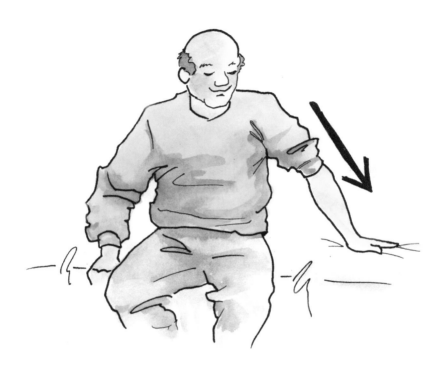

Patient: Shift weight onto your weak arm. Keep your elbow straight, and repeat on your other arm.

Shifting Weight onto the Weak Side

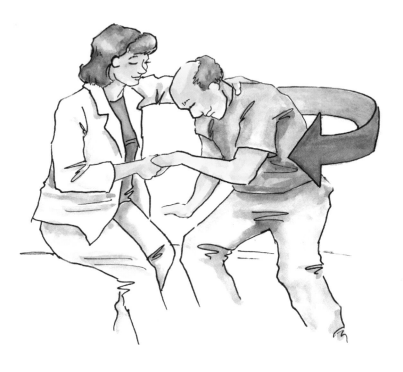

Caregiver: Using a circular motion, help the patient shift weight onto the weak side. Repeat on the strong side.

Patient: Try to put weight onto your weak side.

Preparing to Stand

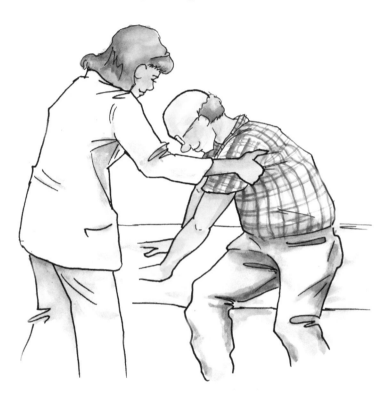

Caregiver: Shift the patient's weight onto both hands, elbows, shoulders, right hip, and right leg by holding lightly onto the patient's arm.

Patient: Shift weight onto both of your arms.

Standing Up

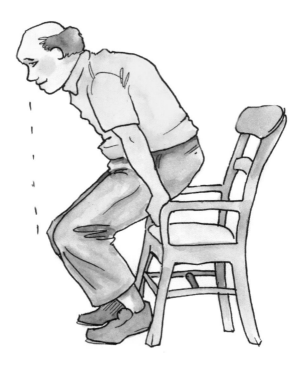

Patient: Shift your weight forward. Align your nose with your
knees. Put your hands on the arm rests for safety.

Preparing for Transfer – Rocking

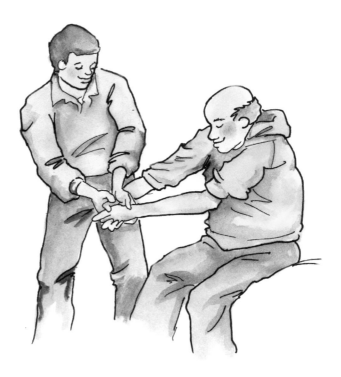

Caregiver: Hold the patient's hands and pull gently forward.

Patient: Pull your head forward. This can be done by rocking forward and backward to allow your body to learn the motion.

Transferring from Wheelchair to Bed

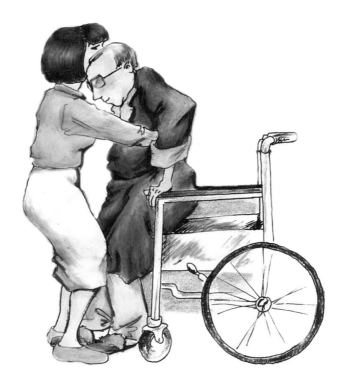

Caregiver: Support the patient and direct the body movement forward (keep your knees bent to alleviate back strain).

Patient: Push with both hands, and move your head forward.

Walking with the Patient

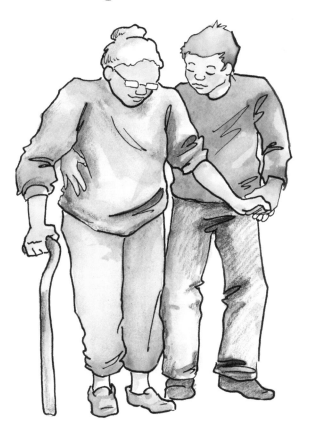

Caregiver: Stand on the patient's weak side and provide support. Do not push.

Patient: Shift your weight to one leg before lifting your other leg.

Using a Walker

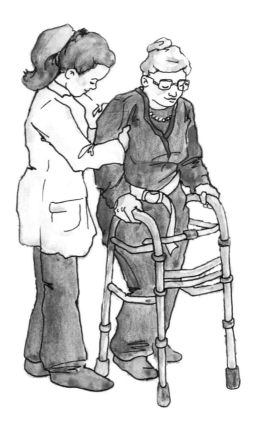

Caregiver: Support the patient's body from the weak side.

Patient: Put both hands on the walker, and shift weight onto your hands when moving your weak leg forward.

Regaining the Use of Hands

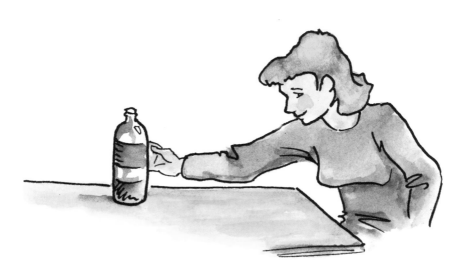

Patient: Practice reaching for familiar objects with one hand at a time. Breathe out when you reach forward, and breathe in when you straighten up.

Moving Both Hands

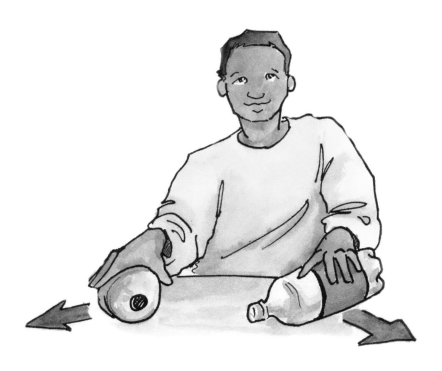

Patient: Hold two bottles, and roll them from right to left, and forward and backward.

Standing on the Weak Side

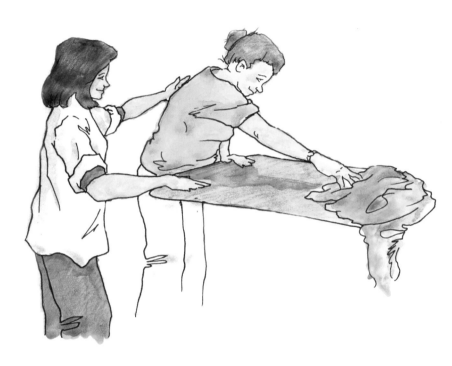

Patient: Stand with equal weight on both of your legs, and provide support by using your good hand.

Caregiver: Stand on the patient's weak side to give help as needed.

High-level Balancing for Upper Body

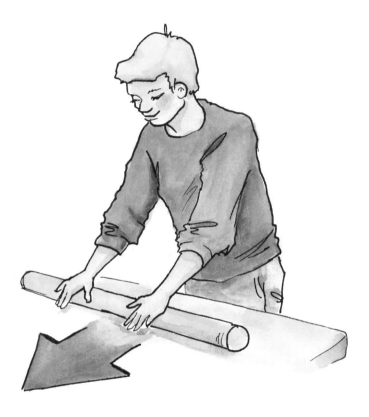

Patient: Stand up near a stable desk, and roll an object on the surface with both of your hands.

Higher-level Dynamic Balancing

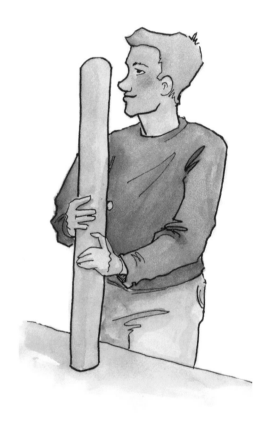

Patient: Stand up near a stable desk. Hold a round, long object upright, and move your arms up and down.

High-level Balancing for Lower Body

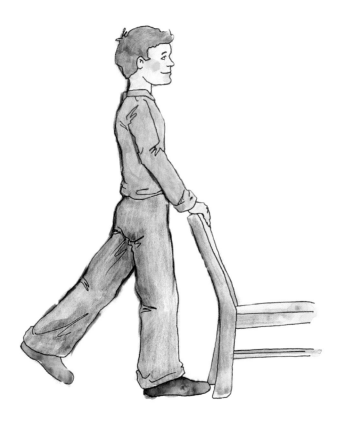

Patient: Hold onto a chair or parallel bars, and pull one leg backward to strengthen your back and leg.

Very High-level Balancing

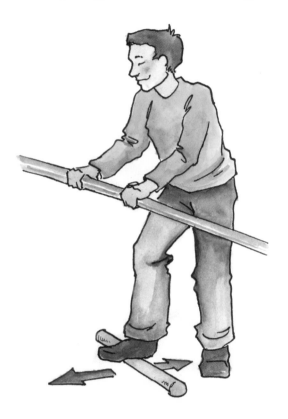

Patient: Hold onto a bar with both hands. With one foot, roll a round stick forward and backward.

Support and Online Resources

These resources can help you and your loved ones deal with the effects of a stroke.

American Heart Association
www.americanheart.org

American Occupational Therapy Association
www.aota.org

American Physical Therapy Association
www.apta.org

American Speech-Language-Hearing Association
www.asha.org/public/speech/disorders/Stroke.htm

American Stroke Association
www.strokeassociation.org

Harvard Health Publications/Harvard Medical School
www.health.harvard.edu./special_health_reports/Stroke.htm

Internet Stroke Center
www.strokecenter.org

Medicare Information Source
www.medicare.org

Medifocus
www.medifocus.com

National Aphasia Association
www.aphasia.org

National Easter Seal Society
www.easterseals.com

National Institute of Neurological Disorders and Stroke
www.ninds.nih.gov

National Stroke Association
www.stroke.org
800-787-6537

Rosalynn Carter Institute for Caregiving
www.rci.gsw.edu

Stroke Awareness for Everyone (SAFE)
www.strokesafe.org

Stroke Clubs International
www.ninds.nih.gov/find_people/voluntary_orgs/volorg217.htm

Stroke Help
www.strokehelp.com

Well Spouse Association
www.wellspouse.org

William Beaumont Hospital Stroke Center
www.beaumonthospitals.com/strokecenter

References

Bach-Y-Rita, Paul. "Brain Plasticity as a Basis for Recovery of Function in Humans." *Neuropsychology* 28 (1990): 547–553.

Bobath, Bertha. *Adult Hemiplegia: Evaluation and Treatment.* London: William Heinman Books, 1978.

Bohannon, Richard W. "Lateral Trunk Flexion Strength: Impairment, Measurement Reliability and Implications Following Unilateral Brain Lesion." *International Journal of Rehabilitation Research* 15, no. 3 (1992): 249–251.

Caleffi, Paula, A. Segura, S. Veloso Fontes, M. Maiumi Fukujima, and S. L. de Andrade Matas. "The Impact Evaluation of Physical Therapy on the Quality of Life of Cerebrovascular Stroke Patients." *International Journal of Rehabilitation Research* 29, no. 3 (2006): 243–246.

Church, C., C. Price, A. D. Pandyan, S. Huntley, R. Curless, and H. Rodgers. "Randomized Controlled Trial to Evaluate the Effect of Surface Neuromuscular Electrical Stimulation to the Shoulder After Acute Stroke." *Stroke* 37, no. 12 (2006): 2995–3001.

Davies, Patricia M. *Steps to Follow.* New York: Springer-Verlag, 1994.

Donnelly, M., M. Power, M. Russell, and K. Fullerton. "Randomized Controlled Trial of an Early Discharge Rehabilitation Service: The Belfast Community Stroke Trial." *Stroke* 35, no. 1 (2004): 127–133.

Dvir, Z., and E. Panturin. "Measurement of Spasticity and Associated Reactions in Stroke Patients Before and After Physiotherapeutic Intervention." *Clinical Rehabilitation* 7, no. 1 (1993): 15–21.

Edmans, J. A., J. R. Gladman, S. Cobb, A. Sunderland, T. Pridmore, D. Hilton, and M. F. Walker. "Validity of a Virtual Environment for Stroke Rehabilitation." *Stroke* 37, no. 11 (2006): 2770–2775.

Embrey, D. G., L. Yates, and D. H. Mott. "Effects of Neuro-Developmental Treatment and Orthoses on Knee Flexion During Gait Single-Subject Design." *Physical Therapy* 70, no. 1 (1990): 626–637.

Fritz, S. L., A. L. Pittman, A. C. Robinson, S. C. Orton, and E. D. Rivers. "An Intense Intervention for Improving Gait, Balance, and Mobility for Individuals with Chronic Stroke: A Pilot Study." *Journal of Neurologic Physical Therapy* 31, no. 2 (2007): 71–76.

Hesse, S. A., M. T. Jahnke, C. M. Bertelt, C. Schreiner, D. Lucke, and K. H. Mauritz. "Gait Outcome in Ambulatory Hemiparetic Patients After a 4-Week Comprehensive Rehabilitation Program and Prognostic Factors." *Stroke* 25, no. 10 (1994): 1999–2004.

Katz-Leurer, M., I. Sender, O. Keren, and Z. Dvir. "The Influence of Early Cycling Training on Balance in Stroke Patients at the Sub-Acute Stage. Results of a Preliminary Trial." *Clinical Rehabilitation* 20, no. 5 (2006): 398–405.

Klein-Vogelbach, Susanne. *Functional Kinetic in Therapeutic Exercise.* New York: Springer-Verlag, 1992.

Lamontagne, A., and J. Fung. "Faster Is Better: Implications for Speed-intensive Gait Training After Stroke." *Stroke* 35, no. 11 (2004): 2543–2548.

Langhammer, B., and J. K. Stanghelle. "Bobath or Motor Relearning Programme? A Comparison of Two Different Approaches, Physiotherapy in Stroke Rehabilitation: A Randomized Controlled Study." *Clinical Rehabilitation* 14, no. 4 (2000): 361–369.

Lannin, N. A., A. Cusick, A. McCluskey, and R. D. Herbert. "Effects of Splinting on Wrist Contracture After Stroke: A Randomized Controlled Trial." *Stroke* 38, no. 1 (2007): 111–116.

Laufer, Y. "The Effect of Walking Aids on Balance and Weight-bearing Patterns of Patients with Hemiparesis in Various Stance Positions." *Physical Therapy* 83, no. 2 (2003): 112–122.

Lennon, S. "Gait Re-education Based on the Bobath Concept in Two Patients with Hemiplegia Following Stroke." *Physical Therapy* 81, no. 3 (2001): 924–935.

Liepert, J., H. Gauder, H. R. Wolfgang, W. H. Miltner, E. Taub, and C. Weiller. "Treatment-induced Cortical Reorganization After Stroke in Humans." *Stroke* 31, no. 6 (2000): 1210–1216.

McCain, K. J., and P. S. Smith. "Locomotor Treadmill Training with Body-Weight Support Prior to Over-Ground Gait: Promoting Symmetrical Gait in a Subject with Acute Stroke." *Top Stroke Rehabilitation* 14, no. 5 (2007): 18–27.

Miller, E. W., M. E. Quinn, and P. G. Seddon. "Body Weight Support Treadmill and Over Ground Ambulation Training for Two Patients with Chronic Disability Secondary to Stroke." *Physical Therapy* 82, no. 1 (2002): 53–61.

Montgomery, Jacqueline, ed. *Physical Therapy for Traumatic Brain Injury.* New York: Churchill Livingstone, 1995.

Mudie, M. H., U. Winzeler-Mercay, S. Radwan, and L. Lee. "Training Symmetry of Weight Distribution After Stroke: A Randomized Controlled Pilot Study Comparing Task-related Reach, Bobath, and Feedback Training Approaches." *Clinical Rehabilitation* 16, no. 6 (2002): 582–592.

Nudo, Ralph J., Birute M. Wise, Frank SiFuentes, and Garrett W.

Millikent. "Neural Substrates for the Effects of Rehabilitation Training on Motor Recovery After Ischemic Infarct." *Science*, no. 272 (June 21, 1996): 1791–1794.

Nudo, Randolph J., W. M. Jenkins, M. M. Merzenich, T. Prejean, and R. Grenda, "Neurophysiological Correlates of Hand Preference in Primary Motor Cortex of Adult Squirrel Monkeys." *The Journal of Neuroscience* 12, no. 8 (August 1992): 2918–2947.

Page, S. J., and P. Levine. "Modified Constraint-induced Therapy in Patients with Chronic Stroke Exhibiting Minimal Movement Ability in the Affected Arm." *Physical Therapy* 87, no. 7 (2007): 872–878.

U.S. Department of Health and Human Services. *Medicare Part B Reference Manual.*

Van der Lee, J. H., R. C. Wagenaar, G. J. Lankhorst, T. W. Vogelaar, W. L. Deville, and L. M. Bouter. "Forced Use of the Upper Extremity in Chronic Stroke Patients: Results from a Single-Blind Randomized Clinical Trial." *Stroke* 30, no. 11 (1999): 2369–2380.

Verrill, D., C. Barton, W. Beasley, and W. M. Lippard. "The Effects of Short-term and Long-term Pulmonary Rehabilitation on Functional Capacity, Perceived Dyspnea, and Quality of Life." *Chest* 128, no. 2 (2005): 673–683.

Winstein, Carolee J., Elizabeth R. Gardner, Donald R. McNeal, Patricia S. Barto, and Diane E. Nicholsen. "Standing Balance Training: Effect on Balance and Locomotion in Hemiparetic Adult." *Archive Physical Medicine Rehabilitation* 70 (October 1989): 755–762.

About the Author

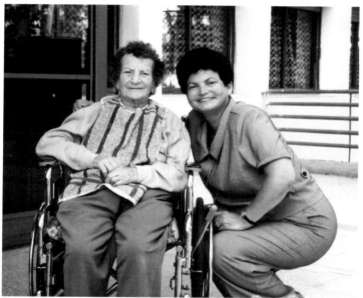

Yaffa Liebermann with her mother, Rachel Steinman, after her mother suffered from a brain attack.

Yaffa Liebermann graduated in 1966 from the Asaf-Arofa school of physiotherapy, which is affiliated with Tel Aviv University in Israel. She served as a physical therapist in the IDF forces during the 1967 war, where she gained experience treating war-related injuries—like amputations, head trauma, and burns—from both sides of the fence. She was shocked to learn and realize how devastating the long-standing results of a war could be. Her varied experience covered positions at an acute hospital, orthopedic clinic, psychiatric clinic, home care, and sub-acute unit for spinal cord injury and head trauma. She has worked in Israel, Switzerland, and the USA.

In 1996 she founded Prime Rehabilitation Services, Inc., which provides physical, occupational, and speech rehabilitation services to sub-acute nursing home facilities throughout the tri-state area: New Jersey, New York, and Pennsylvania.

Yaffa is a certified neuro-developmental therapist (NDT) in adult hemiplegia. She has developed mastectomy and pulmonary rehabilitation programs that were implemented in both hospitals and respiratory centers. She found her love and passion working with the elderly in the nursing home environment. She's a geriatric clinical specialist (GCS), board certified by the American Physical Therapy Association (APTA).

Yaffa is the geriatric liaison for the APTA of New Jersey, and she serves on the Education and Best Practice Committees of the Health Care Association of New Jersey. She lectures to therapists, nurses, caregivers, and family members on ways to improve care for patients. Topics include proper breathing, wellness exercises, proper body mechanics, and stroke restoration, amongst others. Yaffa hopes to educate people about how patients can breathe better and perform movements in a safe and correct way—so they can prevent future injuries and carry their bodies in a healthy and beautiful way.

About Prime
Rehabilitation Services

Prime Rehabilitation Services, Inc. (PRS) is a comprehensive support network of experienced professional physical therapists, occupational therapists, and speech language pathologists who create a complete and continuous program of individualized therapy to improve the quality of life for nursing home residents. Our executive staff has over fifty years of experience in therapy, business management, and administration, providing the highest quality of services in their respective fields. They personally visit each facility on a regular basis to ensure a high level of customer satisfaction and the continuation of our great program.

PRS hires therapists who love to treat the elderly with a soft and caring touch. They encourage patients to excel and achieve the highest possible level of functional independence. PRS provides a pleasant work environment that resonates well with therapists. Company social events, quarterly education sessions, and off-site training activities all contribute to the high employee retention level.

Each facility's director of rehabilitation focuses on overseeing the program, the therapists, and billing management. He or she communicates regularly with all department heads to ensure that PRS becomes an integral part of patient care.

PRS has a deep understanding of PPS (prospective payment system) billing, and we have developed a comprehensive and unique therapy system that includes capturing the appropriate PPS categories, treating long-term residents, and establishing effective relationships with HMOs. Medicare regulations for therapists and licensing regulations change almost daily. PRS is constantly creating and revising proprietary paperwork. We immediately respond to and address all Medicare reviews and denials. We understand billing rule systems, and we make changes as appropriate to counteract any downward trends and assist the patient's progress.

Education is one of our top priorities. We are actively involved in the resident's discharge planning process, and provide education sessions for the therapists and nursing staff, updating them on topics such as prospective payment systems (PPS), minimum date set (MDS), restorative nursing, Medicare documentation, ergonomics, and billing compliance.

As a company, we do what it takes to support our therapists "behind the scenes" so they will be able to provide great care to the patients.

Prime Rehabilitation Services, Inc.

(732) 493-3100   www.primerehab.com
Fax (732) 493-4285   info@primerehab.com

Printed in the United States
140156LV00001BA